Lifestyle Fitness

The Average Person's Guide to a Happier, Healthier, and Fulfilled Life

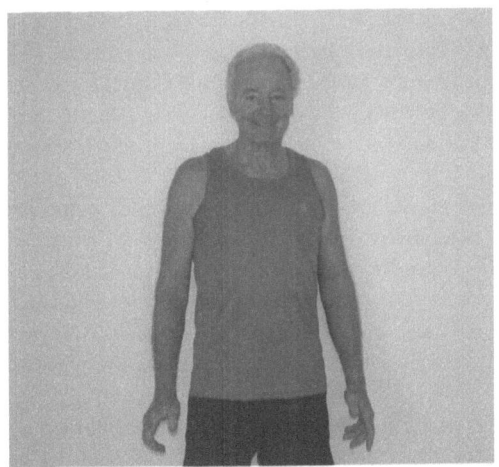

ROBERT NEEVES

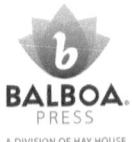

BALBOA.
PRESS

A DIVISION OF HAY HOUSE

Balboa Press books may be ordered through booksellers or by contacting:

Balboa Press
A Division of Hay House
1663 Liberty Drive
Bloomington, IN 47403
www.balboapress.com.au
1 (877) 407-4847

Because of the dynamic nature of the Internet, any web addresses or links contained in this book may have changed since publication and may no longer be valid. The views expressed in this work are solely those of the author and do not necessarily reflect the views of the publisher, and the publisher hereby disclaims any responsibility for them.

The author of this book does not dispense medical advice or prescribe the use of any technique as a form of treatment for physical, emotional, or medical problems without the advice of a physician, either directly or indirectly. The intent of the author is only to offer information of a general nature to help you in your quest for emotional and spiritual well-being. In the event you use any of the information in this book for yourself, which is your constitutional right, the author and the publisher assume no responsibility for your actions.

Any people depicted in stock imagery provided by Thinkstock are models, and such images are being used for illustrative purposes only.
Certain stock imagery © Thinkstock.

Print information available on the last page.

ISBN: 978-1-5043-0219-7 (sc)
ISBN: 978-1-5043-0220-3 (e)

Balboa Press rev. date: 04/26/2016

CONTENTS

ACKNOWLEDGEMENT

I would like to thank my wife Trish for sitting at the computer for many hours turning my hand written scribble into the finished work. My daughter Nicole and her husband Chris for assisting with the exercise images in the book and Leisa for the image quality.

ABOUT THE AUTHOR

My name is Robert Neeves. I am a seventy-year-old personal trainer.

When I was twelve years of age, I contracted rheumatic fever. I was unable to walk and was bedridden for six months. Not wanting to let this affect my life, I put all my energy into my recovery, and at the age of fourteen, after a lot of determination on my part, I became Cronulla De La Salle College Under-Fifteen Athletic Champion. Rheumatic fever also left me with a heart murmur, which made me unable to pass the physical for military service during the Vietnam War.

I have been playing competition squash for close to fifty years. I still compete. Although my reaction time has slowed a little, my movement around the court is still good. I attribute this to my daily exercise routine.

At age sixty-nine I successfully climbed Mount Kilimanjaro-Tanzania. I reached the highest peak of 5,895 metres.

Most of my working life I spent working as a motor mechanic. After retiring at the age of sixty-five, I read an article in the local paper about a personal trainer who was disabled. His story inspired me to achieve my goal of becoming an exercise professional.

I am a registered exercise professional with Fitness Australia (registration number 058426). My specializations include:

Gym instructor

Personal trainer

Older adults' trainer

Children's trainer

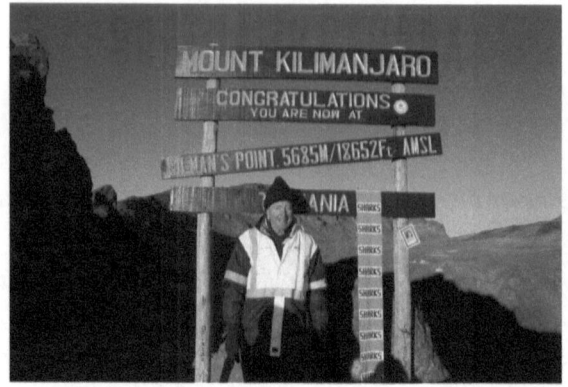

DEPARTMENT OF LABOUR AND NATIONAL SERVICE

Mr. Robert M. Neeves

381 Port Hacking Road,

CARINGBAH   N.S.W.

National Service Registration Office,
Commonwealth Centre,
Elizabeth Street,
SYDNEY. N.S.W.

Registration No. 1005740

23rd July, 1965

Dear Sir,

    I am writing to tell you that you do not meet the standards of fitness required of persons called upon to render service under the National Service Act.

    You should preserve this letter carefully in case it should be necessary to produce it at any time as evidence that you are not required for service.

        Yours faithfully,

        Registrar

NS 14A (Rev 5/65)

D.L.S.C. CRONULLA.
Athletics Champion.
Under 15.
1960
R. NEEVES.

Trophies by : G. B. STAUNTON
335 ILLAWARRA ROAD, MARRICKVILLE   LL 5961

INTRODUCTION

This book, I hope, will enhance the lives of many people of all age groups. I hope you will use it to improve yourself and your lifestyle with moderate, regular exercise. If you are already active and playing some type of sport, hopefully a regular exercise program will make that and any other activity more enjoyable. You do not have to be a fanatic or practically kill yourself every time you work out, but you do have to be consistent and train on a regular basis three or four times a week, preferably with a day off in between. This will help to maintain or improve your current well-being for as long as possible. It's no good having a long life if you cannot enjoy it and spend more time with friends and family. Getting a good night sleep is very important. While you are sleeping your body will repair itself.

If your doctor approves it as okay with any current medication you may be taking, try having a mini fast as often as possible. It is usually easiest to achieve this during the week. If you finish your evening meal by around seven o'clock, do not have any solid food until breakfast. Remember to keep well hydrated and take any medication as prescribed. By doing this, you can achieve a ten- to twelve-hour fast on a regular basis while you sleep. Intermittent fasting, when used sensibly, can aid in weight loss. It will give your digestive system a rest, and it also energizes your metabolism to burn fat. It can also help regulate your eating patterns and help anyone with binge eating disorders. How long is it since your body has had a rest from constant food intake?

Do not set yourself yo-yo goals—up one day down the next. Make slow, gradual, long-term, moderate changes that you can easily sustain. It is important to give your body time to adjust.

Try to get into an 80/20 routine. Practice your new lifestyle changes during 80 percent of your time. Give yourself small treats, have a night out, relax, and enjoy yourself during 20 percent of your time. The 20 percent will help you achieve your 80 percent goals. Try to put some balance into your life.

Be positive about your ageing. Don't think old – think young! Have a whole new attitude to life. Give your life a sense of purpose. Stay mentally strong and do things that make your life worthwhile. Don't sit around and count the days; try to make every day interesting.

Don't hold a grudge, even if you feel its justified. Don't allow others to bring you down. Don't waste time worrying about anything that is out of your control and that you cannot change. Put your everything into making the best of every situation. Do your own thing and believe in yourself. Remember, the only time you fail at something in life is when you stop trying. Most happy people have clear-cut goals. You should wake up each morning in this frame of mind.

PREVENTION IS BETTER THAN CURE—INVEST IN YOUR LIFE!

During our lifetimes, we pay for health, job, and life insurance so we won't become a burden to our families as we grow older. Try looking at your active lifestyle as you would your superannuation fund: you pay a small amount over a long period to gain a large benefit, right? Investing some of your time in an exercise program will cost little, but the benefit to your overall health will be great. Missing an exercise session is like missing a payment into your super account; there are still benefits as long as you do not stop completely. Remember, it is never too late to start. Over thousands of years, our bodies evolved by working hard so we could feed ourselves and avoid danger. Human beings were not meant to be sitting at a desk all day or engaging in other inactive pastimes; we *need* to add exercise to our daily routine.

It's hard to think of an activity in life that cannot be improved upon or made easier by regular exercise.

Compare your body to a tree: your arms are the branches, your core is the trunk, and your legs and feet are the roots. For a tree to be healthy, all three areas need to be in good condition. Your body is no different, so when possible, exercise your whole body.

As we age, our balance becomes incredibly important, as injuries from falls are a major problem. Many falls are preventable. Our best defence is to increase our stability with regular exercise.

Try this simple balance-building exercise: stand on one leg like a stork (use a chair for balance to begin with, if necessary). Try doing this at regular intervals as you gain strength. You can practise while you wait for the kettle to boil!

Sleep

A good, regular night's sleep is important to your overall well-being. Without it, you will not wake refreshed and ready for the full day ahead.

Try to go to bed with as little stress on your mind as possible. Because being tired can magnify a problem, try to sleep with the knowledge that you have done all you can for today. Tomorrow will bring new opportunities.

Whenever possible, set a pattern for the time you sleep. Example plan to go to sleep at 10:00 p.m., and then sleep for eight hours. One hour before bedtime, start to prepare for sleep by shutting down all unnecessary technology like mobile phones, computers and intense television programs. Instead, seek out other forms of lighted entertainment. Read a book, listen to soothing music or watch light, relaxing television. Do all you can to associate your bedroom with relaxation only. This means no computers, phones, or televisions.

Avoid food and alcohol during your preparation period. To avoid becoming dehydrated during the night, make your last alcoholic drink for the night the one you enjoyed with your evening meal

If you need an afternoon nap, take it early, and make it a short one (no more than twenty minutes).

Try relaxing with soft music as you focus on your breathing. Slow, intentional breathing and meditation can help prepare your body for sleep. If you still feel deprived of sleep, have a talk with your healthcare practitioner.

Your Exercise Program Has to Be Your Lifestyle and a Hobby

Don't make exercise something you *have to do*; make it something you *want to do*. Being active can be fun! Your mind-set should be on long-term behaviour change, not short-term, unsustainable success. Getting fit does take time, so make it your passion *and be persistent.* You don't have to be a fanatical or professional athlete to enjoy training to improve your life. Don't think you are fitter than you are; start off slowly. Don't push yourself too hard, too early. Slowly build up your capabilities and let your body be the judge. Set realistic limitations.

Your Eating Habits Have to Be Common Sense

For your body to run at optimal levels, you should reduce your salt, sugar, and fat intake, and reduce your meal size. You do need salt, sugar, and fat in your diet, but not the huge amounts we are consuming in our modern-day lifestyles. Too much of a good thing can be dangerous in the long term. The average person with no serious medical problems should be able to cut out all added salt and sugar. Most "processed" products available at the supermarket (outside of meats and fresh fruits and vegetables) feature added salt, sugar, and fat; the salt (sodium) and sugar included in these products is usually enough for your daily requirements.

It will take time for your body—and particularly, your taste buds—to adjust. Salt, sugar, and fat are not easy to moderate; it will take strong willpower and disciplined self-control to resist the urge to consume all three, but after a month or more, you should not notice the difference in your diet. Your taste will return to normal, and the cravings will not be so strong. Natural food won't taste so bland. You will be eating food that is more beneficial to your body. Be glad of the changes you have made and grateful for the long-term benefits a healthy diet will have on your well-being.

Forget the word *diet*. A diet is a short-term and often unsustainable fix. Instead, create and maintain healthier eating habits that can be sustained over the long term. Be patient! Safe, healthy, and sustainable weight loss can be as little as a half kilo (about a pound) per week. Losing weight slowly gives your body time to adjust to the loss. It also greatly increases your chances of keeping the weight off. Enjoy your food, but don't let food control your life. Being overweight should not become the new norm.

Disclaimer: Before starting any exercise or weight-reducing program, you should consult your healthcare professional, even if you are not overweight and are feeling good. You will be putting your body under more stress than normal. Even though these changes can have great, long-term benefits, you need to rule out any hidden dangerous medical problems before you begin.

Tips on Reducing Salt, Sugar, and Fat

Salt: Use natural herbs and spices instead of adding salt. When shopping, check food labels so you can select products low in sodium (salt), preferably with a content fewer than 120 milligrams of salt per 100 grams of food product. When buying vegetables, commit to buying only fresh or fresh-frozen. Avoid pre-packaged vegetables with added sauces or seasoning. Once your preference for salt has been reduced, you will find it difficult to eat packet chips and the like; they will taste too salty for your new palate.

Sugar: Have sugar-laden drinks only as a social treat. Add honey, berries, and fruit where you would normally add sugar. Honey has about the same calories per serving as sugar, but is more natural. Reduction of sugars is key to your success.

Fat: Trim all fat from meat, and cook on a grill so excess fat can drain away. Choose from lean meats; poultry and fish are ideal. My favourite is turkey steaks. The texture is close to that of red meat, and because you can use similar cooking methods, ground turkey is an ideal replacement for ground beef. Limit your portion size to roughly the size of the palm of your hand. Avoid eating chicken or turkey skin.

Processed Food: Try to eliminate as much heavily processed food from your diet as possible. It lacks nutrients and is quite often packed with salt, sugar, and fat for taste appeal. Always read the labels on food packaging for fat, salt, and sugar content. When you plan your meals ahead of time, you are less likely to stray from your goal.

MOTIVATION

Fear Is a Great Motivator!

What are you most afraid of?
- Developing heart problems, type-2 diabetes, or high blood pressure?
- Developing fatty tissue around your major organs?
- Losing some of your bone density?
- Becoming old before your time?

What are you most afraid of losing?
- Your coordination and reflexes?
- Your muscle tone and strength?
- Your brain function? (Tip: Regular exercise has been known to improve brain function.)
- Your flexibility and pain-free movement?
- Your balance?
- Your looks?
- Your ability to ability to wear all the latest fashions?
- Your disease-free life?

Are You Ready to Enjoy These Benefits of Good Health?
- The feel-good hormones that exercise releases into your body
- Improvement of brain function and hand/eye coordination
- The freedom of movement
- A better life in general
- Reduced stress levels
- Improvement in circulation
- Flexibility in movement

Are You Ready to Become a Good Role Model for Your Family?

Now that you have identified what motivates you, get moving. Don't try to use excuses like some people do.

A friend of mine once told me, "I take a blood-pressure tablet first thing every morning and a cholesterol tablet at night, so I can eat whatever I like and do not have to exercise." I tried to convince him that it doesn't exactly work that way. Maybe sometime in the future we will have a magic tablet to cure all our ailments, but in the meantime, we have to work hard to complement and reduce our reliance on such medications.

Don't avoid starting a training program because of your anxiety about how hard an exercise may be. Avoidance is the easy way out, but it does not have to be complicated. If you follow my guidelines, you will overcome your fears. "Start off slow and keep on the go," I say! No one is going to do the hard work for you. Self-improvement can only come from within yourself. Don't hold back. Invest and believe in yourself, because if you don't, who will? Chase your dreams by making all your steps forward ones. Don't let your fears dictate your goals. All you need is perseverance; no one can stop you except yourself. Don't be afraid to start; you won't regret it. Surround yourself with people who are positive. They can help you change your mind-set from "I can't do that" to "I'll give it a try." You may surprise yourself.

First Week

If you are overweight and have not exercised recently, start by going for a walk. Try to walk for just twenty-five to thirty minutes as often as you can; morning and night are ideal. In summertime, it's best to go in cooler hours. In autumn, winter, or spring, a walk is a great way to catch a little sunshine and some free vitamin D. You must be careful, as the sun can still do damage in these seasons. Walking is so natural; it's a great starting point. If you have already achieved this fitness level, jump ahead to my suggestions for your second week.

Enjoy, relax, and clear your mind!

Second Week

If you have access to a swimming pool, walk through in the water at the shallow end. The mild resistance of the water will tone your muscles without the risk of damage. A bicycle ride is also recommended. The road it is too dangerous; use a stationary bicycle or ride in the park. The best piece of equipment of all is a rowing machine on a low resistance; it will work most if not all your major muscle groups in one hit. If you don't have access to these machines, make your walking time more vigorous and longer.

Embrace a new freedom!

Third week

It is time to get serious about your exercising, whether it is walking, bike riding, swimming pool walking, or rowing. Start at a leisurely pace for ten minutes. This is your warm up. If you are walking, increase to a faster rate for five minutes. If you are doing a more strenuous exercise like bike riding or rowing, make it a one-minute increase. This increase will increase your heart rate. Then reduce your workload until your heart rate returns to normal. Repeat this as many times as you feel comfortable with. You must push yourself a little at a time. Remember, this is hard work, but don't make it so difficult that you cannot sustain it.

Congratulations!

You have started a mild form of high-intensity, short-interval training, known as HISI. Your metabolism is starting to fire up and work in your favour. You are starting to burn fat and will do so for hours after you have stopped exercising.

Exercise

There is no reason you cannot start mild exercise in weeks one, two, or three, providing you have been cleared to exercise by your health care provider.

Before you start any exercise program there is one golden rule that should not be broken:

Posture. Posture. Posture.

Also very important are:

Technique, and then reps and sets.

GOOD POSTURE

Posture is the most important element in any form of exercise. If your posture is not good while you are doing a particular exercise, do not continue with that exercise. If you lose your correct posture during exercising, stop! Your body is telling you that you have done enough.

Your posture whilst you are standing must keep your body in alignment. Your bones and joints must be straight. Imagine a straight line running down from your ear to your ankle. Your head is erect. Your chin is up, your shoulders are back and square. Draw your stomach in towards your spine. Keep your knees neutral (not locked) and your feet forward.

To maintain good posture and to improve your balance, you should try to exercise all your muscle groups equally, both anterior (front) and posterior (back). For example, you should exercise your back upper legs (the hamstring group) and front upper legs (quadriceps) equally. Follow this rule for all of your muscle groups.

Do not use good posture only whilst you are exercising; use it every day and make it your lifestyle.

Bad posture can be the cause of back pain, spinal problems, joint pain and degeneration, rounded shoulders, and even a pot belly.

Here is a quick static postural assessment check:

Stand in your bare feet and with your back against a wall (no skirting board if possible). Be sure your head, shoulders, buttocks, and heels all touch the wall. With your feet pointing straight out, you should feel your body weight in your heels and not have a feeling of falling forward. Normal spine alignment has a natural "S" shape curvature. Check the space between the wall and your lower back by sliding your hand into the space, if your knuckles (with your hand flat) fit snugly, your lower back and arch is acceptable; however, if you can pass a closed fist between the space, you could possibly need professional help.

Next, check your shoulders. If the middle of your upper back touches the wall but your shoulders round forward away from the wall, you need to work on exercising your upper back muscles to pull them back. You should also stretch your chest muscles.

Remember, this is a very quick assessment designed to get you thinking and motivated towards a healthier lifestyle. If you have any concerns, please consult your health care professional.

Golden Rule:

Never, ever compromise on good posture or technique.

Technique is the way an exercise is performed correctly. This is also important, but not as important as posture. If you lose posture, technique will also be lost.

Repetition (Reps)

A rep is the number of each particular exercise you do before you pause or stop. This total number is then referred to as a set. For example eight reps might equal one set.

Good Walking Posture

Don't hunch your shoulders or lean forward. Do not overstride. Your first forward foot contact should be with your heel. In other words, you step heel to toe.

Stay upright and avoid looking down. I say *avoid* rather than *don't* because you should be aware of any uneven ground or obstacles that could cause you to fall or stumble.

Don't let your arms be idle. With your shoulders relaxed, bend your arms at 90 degrees. If you wish to avoid looking like a power walker, a 45-degree bend of your arms will present a more relaxed approach. Move your arms in a backward and forward motion at the same speed as you move your legs, but in opposite directions. To add extra benefit to your walk, try using arm or hand weights or walking on hilly terrain.

Try to increase the intensity of your walk beyond "having an amble." It should be fast enough to make a chat difficult, so that you end up doing a bit of huffing and puffing.

ACHIEVING FITNESS AT HOME
No equipment necessary.

Note: With all these exercises gradually increase reps and range of movement.

Tricep Dips

This exercise helps to tighten up your tuck shop arms—the muscle at back of your upper arm.

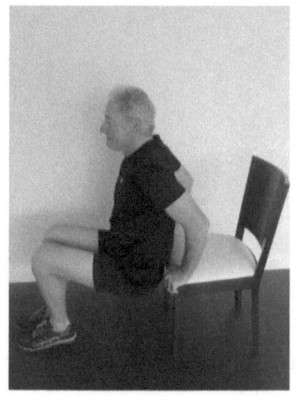

Sit upright on the front edge of a sturdy chair. An unpadded wood or metal straight-back chair works best. Place the palms of your hands next to your backside (glutes) near the edge of the seat. Your knees should form a right angle. Keeping your hands on the chair seat, slide your backside forward off the chair seat, then straight down in front of the chair. Your elbows now form an angle as well. Raise yourself up to the original position. This is one rep. Remember, don't move your body away from the chair; your movement should be straight up and down.

The number of reps you can accomplish will depend on your fitness level. Give your arms a rest. Remember, you can always come back and do more later on. Slowly increase number of reps with each session. The slow increase will prevent muscle soreness and will encourage you to sustain your new lifestyle change.

Chair Squats

Okay, now let's work on your legs. You can do chair squats using same chair.

This is a very effective easy exercise. Sit down about half way back on the chair, keeping your back straight, arms in front, head up and looking forward. Pause for a split second, but do not relax. Keeping your muscles engaged, stand up, driving yourself up through your legs and heels. It is important that you have full heel contact with the floor. When you feel strong enough, do this same exercise without the aid of a chair. You will then be doing "squats."

Leg Extensions

Sit on the chair and move your glutes (backside) back until you are sitting hard against the back of chair. Sit tall so your spine is straight and supported by the back of chair. Place your feet evenly on the floor. Engage your core and raise both legs evenly until they are parallel to the floor. Pause for a few seconds and then slowly lower your legs to the floor, keeping good control of your movement. At first you may grip the side of the chair if necessary for extra control and support. Keep your focus on activating your core during this exercise.

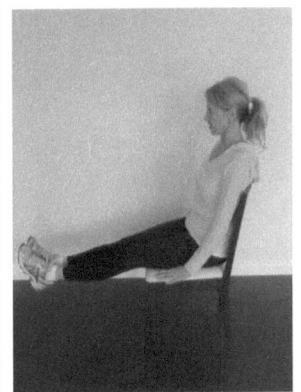

Lunges

This exercise can be done as a static or walking lunge. Assume a good standing posture, take a step forward then drop your body straight down, similar to what you would do showing reverence in a church—genuflect. Your rear knee should almost reach the ground and both legs should form right angles at the knees. Keeping your head up and back straight, push back up to complete one rep. If you need support to keep your balance, place one hand on the back of a chair. Correct technique is straight up, straight down. Do not lean forward. For a static lunge, repeat the exercise on the same spot. For a walking lunge, take successive steps forward.

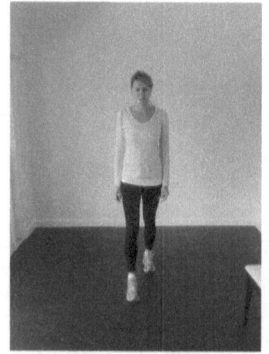 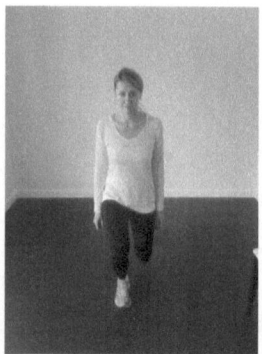 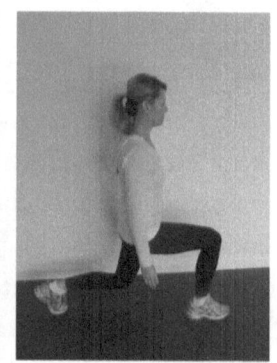

Step ups

If you have steps in your house, always use the bottom step for safety. Using good standing posture, position yourself in front of the step. Begin with either foot. Step up and put your foot on the step. Make sure your foot is wholly on the step. Follow with second foot. Now both feet are completely on the step and you are balanced. Step back down with the same foot you started with. This is one rep. Repeat the rep with opposite foot. Alternate feet as you continue to do reps. This exercise is very simple, but it's great for balance and coordination.

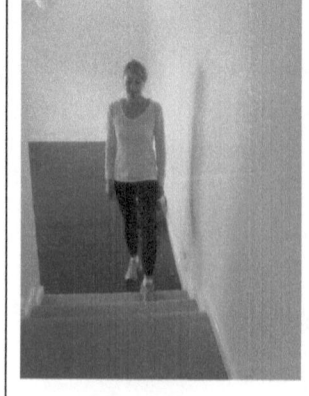

Calf Raises

Use the bottom step once again. With correct standing body posture, stand with both feet on the first step. Only the front half (toes and balls of the feet) are on the step. You heels should be unsupported. Raise and lower your heels, lifting your body weight up and down (not everyone can achieve this). It is okay to raise your arms to keep your balance. It is also okay to hold onto the railing!

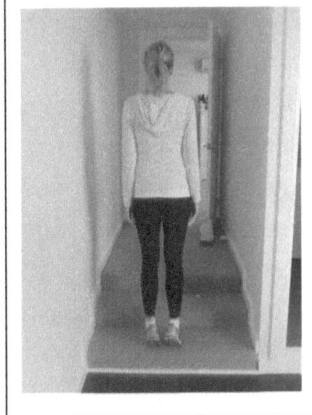

Standing Push Out

This is like a push-up, but you do it standing. Using good standing body posture, stand facing a wall, arm's length away from the wall. Your feet should be shoulder width apart. Reach out and place the palms of your hands on wall. (If it's an interior wall, make sure your hands are clean so you will not leave any marks!) Lower yourself towards the wall until your nose almost touches the wall, then push back. This is one rep.

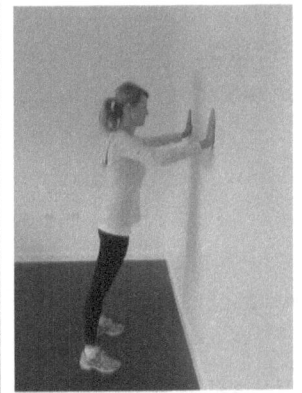

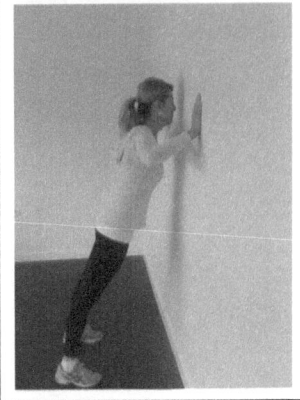

Standing Leg Push Back

This is based on the standing push-out. Still in the same position facing the wall with your hands on the wall, put your feet together, raise your right leg up until it is at a right angle in front of you. Keep your body nice and straight, and keep your arms out straight in front and your hands on wall for balance and support. Without rotating your hips, extend your right leg back, as far and high as you can. Return to starting position and repeat using your left leg. Once you have mastered these two exercises and built up muscles in your arms and legs, try doing push-ups on the floor and while on your knees.

Lateral Arm Raises (Side and Front) with Calf Raises

Maintain good standing body posture. Start with your arms by your side, and raise them out from your side until they reach shoulder height. Do not lock your elbows; keep them slightly bent (this is often called "elbows soft.") Lower your arms back down to your side. Raise them again, but this time straight out in front to shoulder height. Then return them to your side. This is one rep.

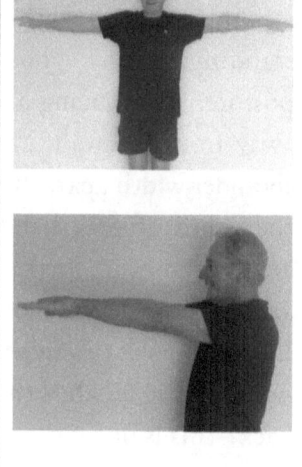

If you want to compound this exercise and get a little more out of it, and your balance is good, combine it with calf raises. As you raise your body by standing on tiptoe, raise and extend your arms alternately between front and side on each calf raise. On front raises, keep arms at shoulder width.

Abdominal Curls / Crunches

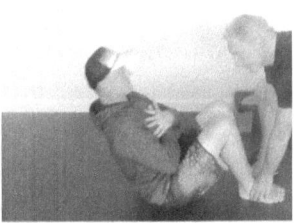

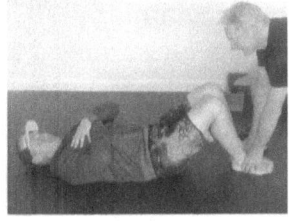

These are commonly known as sit-ups. Sit on the floor with your knees bent and your feet flat on the floor, hip width apart. This will keep your hips square. Your knees should be apart. (I prefer to have my feet locked under a bed frame or lounge chair.) With your back straight and hands across your chest (not behind your head,) engage your abdominal muscles (sometimes know as your six pack), your glutes (the backside muscles), and your hamstring muscles (rear upper leg) and lean back as far as you can feeling confident you will be able to return to a sitting position. Continue to improve your range of movement until your shoulders can rest on the floor and you can return to a straight-up position. If you have your hands behind your head, you may tend to pull your head forward and your chin to your neck. This will result in bad posture and technique. You can also hold your arms out front and slide your hands up your legs.

Opposite Arm, Opposite Leg

This exercise is performed in the dog position. Start on the floor on all fours (hands and knees). Lift your left arm up and straight out in front. Hold for a few seconds then return to all fours. Next lift your right leg straight out to the rear. Again, hold the extension for a few seconds before returning to all fours. Repeat, using the opposite arm and leg. Keep practising this until you are strong enough in your core to hold your opposite arm and leg up together for a few seconds. You will have then achieved a rep. If you are finding it difficult to balance, this is quite normal. Your balance will improve with practice.

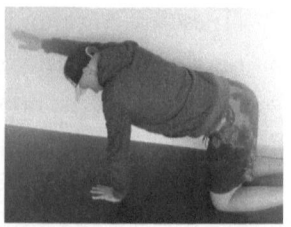

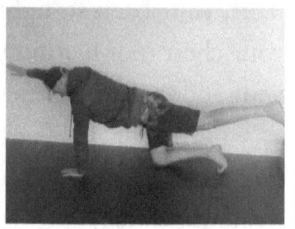

Plank

Start off on the floor on your hands and knees. Engage your core muscles to support your body weight and lower yourself down so you are resting the front part of your body on your elbows and forearms. Holding your hands together, extend one leg back so it is resting on its toes. Do the same with the other leg. You whole body is now supported on your toes, elbows, and forearms. Correct posture is head up, looking at a spot just in front of your hands. Your shoulders to your ankles must resemble a plank (it should be as flat as a board). Keeping those core muscles engaged, hold the position for as long as you can. Do not expect to stay "up" for too long. Even ten seconds is a good start. If you are overweight or not yet very strong, try extending one leg at a time until you become stronger.

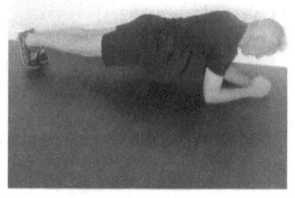

Reverse Crunches

This exercise is more difficult than it looks.

Lie flat on the floor on your back, body fully extended and feet together. Engage your core muscles and then raise both your feet at the same time. Keeping them aligned, hold them approximately 15 to 20 centimetres (6 to 8 inches) off the floor for as long as you can. You should immediately feel your lower abs working overtime. Slowly increase your holding time.

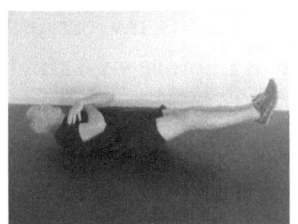

Superman Pose

This is a great exercise for your back, core, and shoulders. Lie on your front side on the floor. Extend your body fully with your arms outstretched in front of your head. You now look the way Superman was depicted in the movies when he was flying, hence the name. Start by lifting one arm at a time, alternating left and right arms. Do the same with your legs. As you progress and get stronger, work up to lifting opposite arm and leg together. This is a back extension exercise and will help balance your exercise program.

Caution! Limit your range of movement to avoid any spine flexion. Add to this exercise by lifting your chest off the ground.

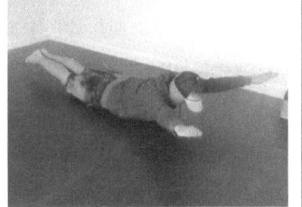

Squats	
This is my favourite exercise. Squats will improve your thighs, hips, and glutes (backside), and will also help to keep your legs in shape. This is the most natural exercise that you can do; in fact, you have been doing it since you were a baby. Some people have forgotten to use it. How do you pick up an item that is below knee height? Most people bend over. No! You should be doing a squat. You have these great, strong lower body muscles, yet you are bending your back. Silly! You can build up to this exercise by using a chair, and then transition to no chair. Stand with your feet the same distance apart as your hips. Form a straight line between your toes, knees, and hips. Engage your abs and slowly lower your body, keeping long in the spine. Go as low as you can while still feeling confident you can raise your body back up. With your head up, drive your body back up through your heels. Keep practising until your knees form a right angle or lower. If you have trouble keeping your balance when you are not using a chair, extend your hands out to the front while focusing on an object that is directly in front of you. Here is a list of tips for perfect squats: • Don't make any side movement; go straight up and down.	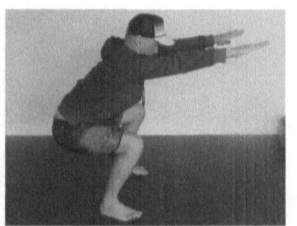

- Stay long in the spine—no hunching.
- Keep your head up and keep looking forward.
- Always keep your heel in contact with floor.
- Draw your belly button to your spine.
- Keep your knees "soft" (slightly bent) at top of movement.
- Breathe in on the down movement and out as you drive back up.
- Extend arms forward for balance.
- Check your form by looking at a mirror that is off to your side.

Knees to Elbows

Stand with feet a little wider apart than your shoulders. With your head up, stand tall. Extend your right arm out in front of you. Your upper arms should form a 90-degree angle with your body, and your elbow should form a 90-degree angle. Raise your left knee up and across to meet your right elbow or as close to it as you can. Ten reps make one set. Next do right knee to left elbow, another ten reps.

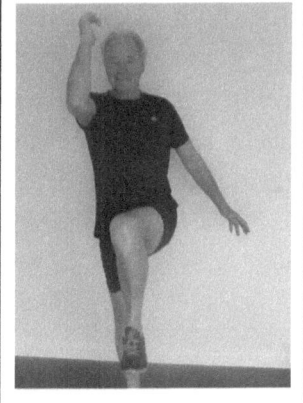

Elbows to Knees

The starting position is the same as it is for knees to elbows. This time do a squat, bringing your right elbow across your body toward your left knee. Push back up to start position then alternate to left elbow to right knee. Do twenty alternating reps to a set.

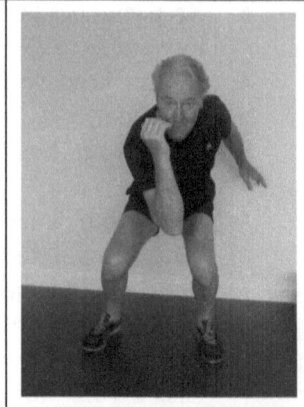

Mountain Climb

Start in full push-up position on floor. Your body weight should be supported by the palms of your hands and your toes. Bring your left knee forward towards your chest, keeping your core tight. Return to the starting position. Repeat with the right knee. This is a difficult exercise, so start with a few reps and slowly build up over time.

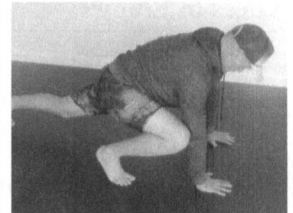

Walkout

With your body in same position you used for mountain cimb, slowly walk hands backwards and forwards. This exercise requires good balance and stability. It's a great core exercise.

Side Step

Keeping a good standing posture, walk across the room sideways: Extend your right foot out to the side and place it on the floor. Bring the left foot up and place it next to the right foot. Continue this way across the room. Lead with your left foot on the way back. Add a squat at each end before returning.

Biceps Curl

Find something around the house that you can hold in two hands that also has a bit of weight to it. A frypan works well, or a heavy broom. While standing tall, hold your chosen object in both hands, palms up, with your arms at full length in front of you so the object is below your waist. Keeping a straight back and with your head up, bend your elbows and curl the object to your chest. Return it to the starting position. This is one rep.

Air Circles

Stand with good body posture, arms extended shoulder height out to the side, perpendicular to your torso. Rotate your arms in opposite directions on a vertical plane. Reverse the motion. This is a great exercise to do at the beginning, in the middle, and at the end of each session. See more information in the next chapter.

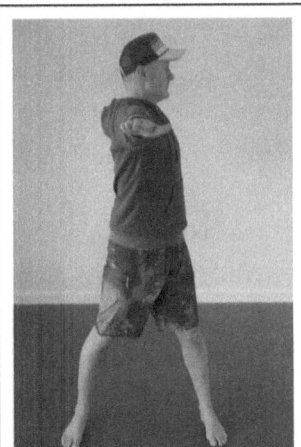

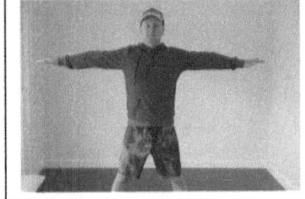

Stretching and Breathing

As you start to increase the length and intensity of your exercise session, it is important to do some stretching before and after more vigorous movement. This will help prevent injuries and some of the stiffness you might experience as a result of your exercises. You should expect some mild stiffness for twenty-four hours after a workout, especially in the first few weeks. This will ease as you build stronger muscles. Remember that, when you are working out, some mild muscle burn is okay. Sharp pain is not! If this should occur, stop immediately.

Dynamic Stretching before Exercise; Static Stretching after Exercise

Dynamic stretching sounds a bit dramatic. In simple terms, it means a slow increase in movement to get your resting muscles ready for exercise by increasing muscle length and blood flow to muscles.

Start with a walk and gradually increase intensity of leg movement. Do the same with your arms. Move them every which way you can think of. Think of the program ahead. Do slow half exercises so you mimic the exercise but limit your range of movement while slowly increasing the range. Do half lunges, squats, arm circles, high knees, and so forth, so you warm up with slow increases in range of movement and intensity to flow and blend into the start of your session.

Static Stretching – After a Hard Work Out

Okay, time to wind down, relax your mind, and commence static stretching, which is the opposite to dynamic stretching

Dynamic = Plenty of movement
Static = Stationary or at rest
The golden rule for static stretching = Tension but no pain

As with dynamic stretching, static stretching requires gradual increases, except this time movement is slow and controlled with low force to allow relaxation. Hold each stretch for approximately five seconds and repeat five times with slow increases. Keep movement controlled. There should be no bouncing and no pain. Most static stretching can be thought of as a movement opposite to how you have been exercising.

BREATHING

Correct breathing is important with any exercise. As you increase the intensity and workload, it becomes even more important.

I have no medical training or evidence that my advice is correct procedure, but it is what I believe works for me.

During rest breaks, take in a deep breaths through your nose and release smaller amounts out through your mouth. We want to expand your lungs with those deep breaths and keep plenty of oxygen in your lungs for your body to use. Muscles need oxygen; lack of it can cause muscles to burn. Try to load up your lungs with air before you need it.

When exercising it is easy to remember: breathe in when load is lightest and out when load is heaviest.

A good example is the squat exercise. When you lower your body down you are working with gravity, but you still need your muscles engaged for control. The load is at its lightest, so take a deep breath. As you drive back up, lifting your body weight against gravity takes a more strenuous effort, so exhale and get ready for next rep.

If you can, raise the intensity of your exercise session so your breathing is heavy enough to experience some slight difficulty in carrying on a normal conversation.

STATIC STRETCHING EXERCISES

Always start with and keep good posture.

If you are restricted from doing these exercises or stretching to the full extent for any reason—illness, injuries, lack of flexibility, or other reason—do whatever you can, any movement is good.

Bicep Stretch	
Standing tall with arms extended out front, rotate hands so your palms are joined and facing each other, one palm facing up and one facing down. Apply pressure with your top hand onto your bottom hand to stretch the lower straight arm.	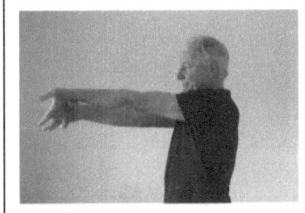

Chest Stretch	
Stand tall with arms extended out to your sides parallel to ground, palms forward (so your look like a cross). Slowly push arms backwards.	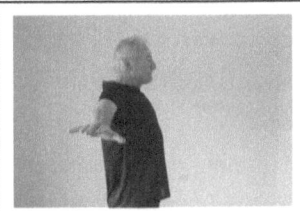

Upper Back Stretch	
Fold your hands together in front of your chest. Turning your gripped hands inside out, and keeping fingers interlaced, stretch your arms out in front of you, shoulder high, pushing away from your chest.	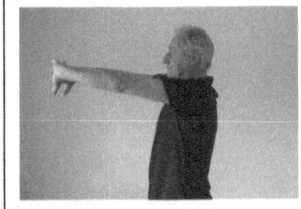

Shoulder/Tricep Stretch

Standing tall, place one hand behind your head so your palm is against your neck. With your other hand, grab your elbow and pull it gently in front of your face.

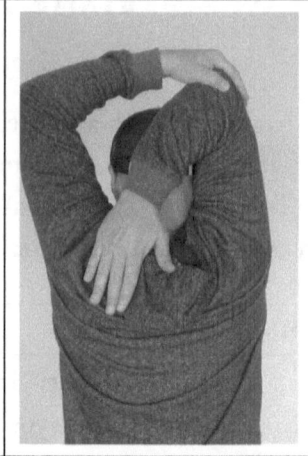

Side Stretch

Stand tall with your feet shoulder width apart, arms at full length resting by your side, with your palms facing towards your body. Without leaning backwards or forwards bend your body to one side, sliding your hand down your leg. Return to a vertical position and then repeat the same bend to the other side.

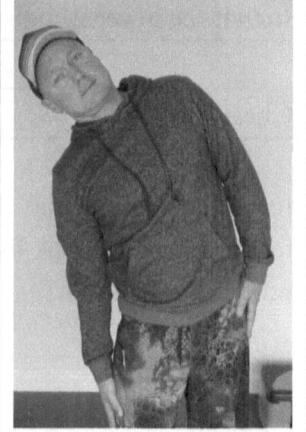

Hip/Thigh Stretch

While standing tall, take a large step forward. Slowly lower your body down just as you would do for a lunge. Use slow, gradual movements and repeat with the opposite leg forward.

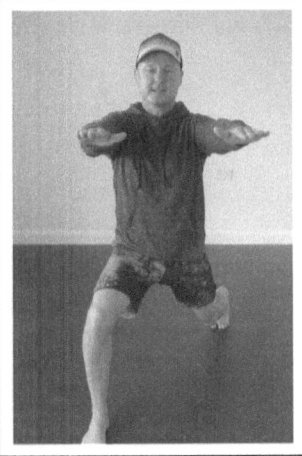

Calf Stretch

While standing in front of a wall, lean towards the wall and place palms of both hands on the wall. Brace yourself the same way you would if you were trying to push the wall over, with one leg bent and one leg straight. The straight leg is the one getting the stretch so swap leg position to complete. Stand as far away from the wall as necessary to feel a good stretch in your calf muscles.

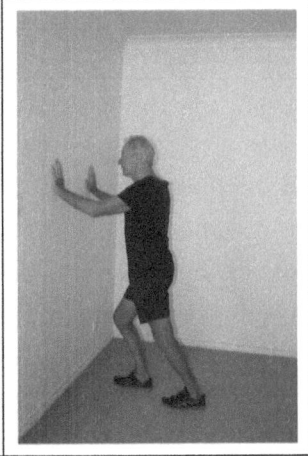

Adductor Stretch (upper inside leg)

Keeping a straight back, stand with your feet wide apart in what we might call a sumo wrestler's stance. Lower your body weight slowly to the right, keeping your right leg bent and your left leg straight. Your left adductor is now being stretched. Repeat on opposite side.

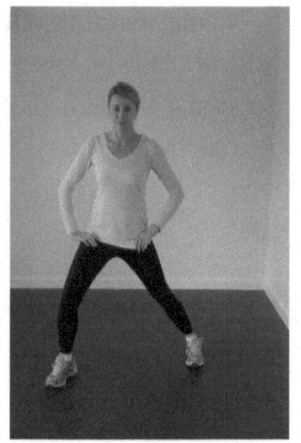

(from this position, lower yourself down)

Groin Stretch

Sit on the floor. Relaxing your knees to the side, keep your back straight and bring the soles of your feet together. Place your hands on your ankles and your elbows on the inside of your knees. Slowly push your knees towards the ground with your elbows.

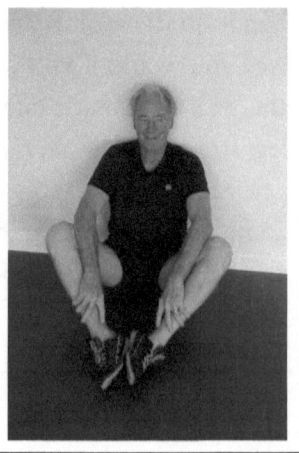

Twist in Seated Position (shoulder, hips, and back)

While sitting on the floor, extend your legs and then bend your right knee so it is pointing up, foot flat on the floor. Place your right foot on the floor against the left side of your left knee. Place your left hand on the floor next to your backside, arm straight. Keeping your right arm straight, place your right elbow against the left side of your right knee. Putting pressure on your right knee with your right arm, twist your torso to the left. Swap your legs and direction to repeat.

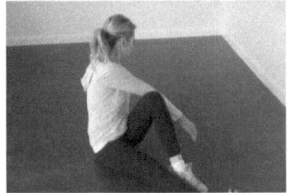

Child Stretch (back and arms)

Sit on your heels, knees together. Lower your chest so it is resting on or close to your knees but still comfortable. Extend your arms in front of you and slowly slide your hand forward on the floor without moving your torso.

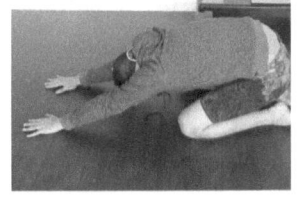

ACTIVE REST

Active rest is a relaxed form of movement to be used in the short breaks between sets in your normal exercise session. You can also use these movements on your recovery days off—those days between hard sessions.

Between exercise sets, keep yourself moving; a short walk as you take in deep breaths can be beneficial for preparing your body for your next set.

On your recovery days, go for a long walk and enjoy the world knowing you have worked hard towards achieving your goals.

Active rest is as important as any exercise session. Start by clearing your mind of any negative thoughts, and try to think of your world as a blank canvas. Relax and take in the sights and sounds of the environment. Whenever possible, leave your phone at home. When your walk is completed, finish with a simple mild stretching routine and slowly return your mind only to the things that are of most importance to you. Try to avoid situations or people that may stress, upset, or drain you. Surround yourself with people who give you energy. Treat your next exercise session like an appointment you do not want to miss.

ANSWER TO A MODERN-DAY PROBLEM

I think the answer to our modern-day obesity problem and sedentary lifestyle is moderate, consistent, long-term exercise. We need to mimic our ancestors who were hunter-gatherers. Their lifestyle, for their entire lives, involved a lot of movement. What a great machine the human body is! And it can take a lot of abuse. But the worst abuse is lack of use.

The human body was designed to do work. In modern days we have all sorts of machines to do that work for us. The muscles we used before machines came along are now going to waste; they have been made redundant. We have removed all of the jobs and tasks that require the need for exertion. That old saying "use it or lose it" is very true.

Leading a sedentary lifestyle, sitting on the lounge for long periods, can make you lethargic and more tired. Getting up and moving, going for a walk, or doing some form of mild exercise can improve your circulation and help reduce stress levels. It also improves your mood and gives you a sense of well-being. Lack of fitness can make easy tasks more difficult. It stands to reason that building up your fitness and muscle mass, even if by only a small amount, may make everyday activity easier and more enjoyable.

Regularity is the key to getting the most benefit out of your exercise program and the new lifestyle it brings about. Four or five sessions of forty-five minutes' duration spread out across the week is of much more benefit than a two-hour session once a week.

Working out consistently and at regular intervals and then giving yourself a good recovery period of twenty-four to forty-eight hours is ideal. This will help you prevent overload and the possibility of losing interest.

Creating a new lifestyle and beginning an exercise program may, for a short period of time, take you out of your comfort zone, but living outside of your comfort zone can be exciting and can give you a new zest for life that will soon become your new norm. Slowly progress in small stages as you move from the new you to an even better you. Remember, slow increases. You must give your body time to adjust. If you want to slow the effect of ageing and avoid premature death plus all the health risks associated with bad health, you have to get off the lounge and *move, move, move!*

ADDING WEIGHT TO YOUR EXERCISE SESSION

Adding free weights to your exercise session is the next move forward. You do not need to use heavy weights to tone and improve muscle strength. With lighter weights, you can do more reps and sets and lessen the chance of injuries.

Weight Selection

Selecting the right size weights to give yourself a great and effective workout, and to avoid injury, can vary depending on the following:

- Body size. A lightly built person will use less weight than someone of a heavier build.
- Male or female. Men, in general, are of a stronger build and can work with heavier weights without fear of injury.
- Intensity of session. As you increase intensity, decrease weight size.
- Fitness level. The more you use your muscles, the stronger you and they get.
- Exercise selected and muscles used. For example, you can use a heavier weight in a bicep curl because the muscle mass is larger and more commonly used. You might choose a lighter weight for a lateral raise because those muscles are not commonly used much in general daily work.

You do not need heavy weights to tone muscles and lose weight. Have fun with plenty of reps and sets. To select the correct weight size and prevent injury choose a weight with which you can do fifteen reps at a leisurely rate with the last three reps becoming a little more difficult. If you can do three sets with a short break in between each set, you have chosen the correct weight. After a few sessions at that weight, try a slight increase in weight. Always remember, however, that posture and technique are paramount as weight increases.

A Great Starting Exercise Kit

Women
- Two 2-kilogram soft weights (The soft weights are kind on your hands.)
- One exercise step

Men
- Two 4-kilogram weights
- One exercise step

You can add weights to some of the exercises previously described. Here are some examples:

- Lunge: Use one weight in each hand at arm's length by your side. Add a bicep curl for a good compound exercise.
- Step up: Start with one weight in each hand, arms down by your side. As you step up, do a bicep curl.
- Abdominal curl: Use one weight held in both hands on your chest.
- Squats: Use one weight held in both hands at chest height.
- Knee to elbows: Hold one weight in each hand, raised to shoulder height.
- Elbow to knee: Hold one weight in each hand, raised to shoulder height.
- High knee: Hold one weight in each hand, raised to shoulder height.
- Bicep curl: Replace household items with weights. You can then use an alternating arm action or both arms together.

Now that you have an exercise step (refer to starting kit), here are two new exercises that will not only improve your fitness and strength, but will also help with your balance and coordination.

Opposite Arm/ Opposite Leg

Stand in front of the step. Step up with your left leg, ensuring that your whole foot is firmly on the step. Follow with right leg, but do not place it on the step. Instead, keep it moving into a high knee position. Do a bicep curl with your left arm so that, at the top of the movement, the opposing arm and leg are raised.

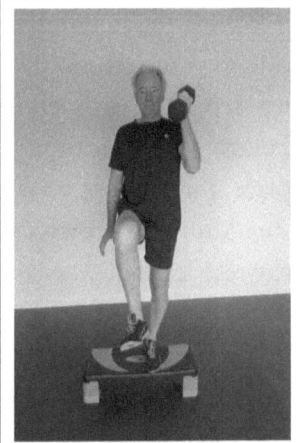

Do ten reps leading with your left leg and ten reps leading with your right leg. Once you have mastered this, try alternating the lead leg after each step, if you find it difficult, you are not alone. Try remembering that the first leg to go up is the same arm that will be raised. Add hand weights and you have a great exercise that is best performed to music. Turn the music up and have fun.

Correct back posture is essential, and it is easy to forget about it when you are concentrating on coordinating your arms and legs.

A variation of this exercise is to hold the full upwards position for a few seconds. You will be standing on one leg with the opposite arm and leg raised. Practise this on the floor before trying it on the step. This is a great exercise for maintaining balance as we age.

Step Across

With the step in front and facing away, approach from rear right side so your left foot is closest to the rear of the step. With your left leg step up so your left foot is firmly on the step but towards the rear. Follow with your right leg, bringing your right foot across and firmly place it in front of your left foot. Step back down on opposite side of step leading with your left leg so as your right foot ends up close to the rear left side, repeat by leading with your right leg to step across.

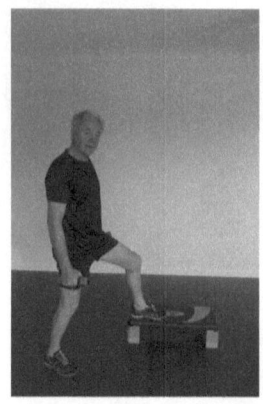 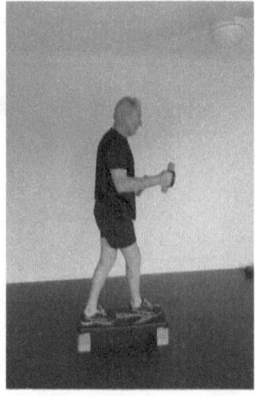 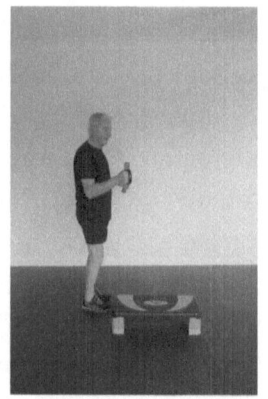

You will notice in the above three images, that my upper body posture is not good.

To Correct ...

1. Lift your shoulders up and push your shoulders back.
2. Lift your head to straighten so your eyes are looking straight ahead.
3. Drop shoulder slightly so they are naturally square.

Working Muscles with Weights

As you add weights to your program, you increase the benefits gained, but you also run the risk of your muscles becoming fatigued, sore, or tight.

Avoiding Sore Muscles

Even though you have been very diligent and have done an intensive static stretching routine after every training session, you may still experience tight or sore muscles for the next twenty-four to forty-eight hours. This is common if you are a beginner or have not trained for a long period. Tight muscles are synonymous with weak muscles. Your muscles are working harder than they are used to. This is not always evident *during* a training session. Unfortunately one size does not fit all, and common sense may be your best guide.

Muscle soreness is not always a good guide to the effectiveness of an exercise program. Even without any post-exercise muscle soreness, you could still be engaging in a good productive program that still gives you scope to make slight increases in weight size and intensity as you move forward. If you do experience soreness that lasts longer than forty-eight hours, you may have sustained an injury. Or it might be that you are working too hard, so you need to ease back on intensity and or weight size or both. Muscles should not feel so tight or sore that they affect your normal activities.

Recovering from Sore Muscles

Stretching is the best way to avoid tight or sore muscles after a hard session of exercise. Do dynamic stretches to warm up before exercising, and static stretches to cool down at the finish. Get plenty of movement (active rest) on your days off between sessions. Movement, even if it is uncomfortable, is better than sitting on the lounge all day. You need to get your circulation moving to help your muscles repair themselves.

Most people enjoy the dynamic stretches leading into more rigorous exercise, but they are less inclined to put time into static stretching, which is just as important. These stretches not only help prevent tight muscular discomfort, they are an additional part of your program and will contribute to the growth of muscle strength, on a smaller scale, because your muscles are still engaged.

You might want to review the static stretches I described in this book; they are that important. Try to think of your static stretches as your muscles stretching in the opposite direction to the direction they stretched during your exercises. You are gradually lengthening the muscles as they cool down slowly, relaxing and returning to your normal range of movement.

Hold each stretch for about five second and repeat it three to five times with small, gradual increases in tension. Remember tension, but no pain.

Whether you have sore muscles or not, a few cups of Epsom salts in a hot bath can work wonders for muscle recovery. It is readily absorbed into the skin and is known to ease mild pain and relieve inflammation.

STRUCTURING YOUR EXERCISE SESSIONS

Any high-energy activity that increases your body temperature should start and finish with hydration.

Hydration: How Water Is Absorbed into Your Body

Your body is 60-65 percent water, so it is important to keep well hydrated. You need to top up your body with about two litres (about eight glasses—eight ounces each) every day, more if you start an exercise program. The first thing you should do every morning is have a glass of water. Continue drinking at regular intervals during the day. A glass every two hours is better than larger amounts at longer intervals.

Consume water before you exercise, and take small amounts regularly during your exercise session, say every fifteen minutes. Don't wait to you feel thirsty and then consume a large amount. Continue your hydration for up to two hours after your session, particularly if you have had a hard sweaty session.

Session Structure

No one exercise program will suit everybody, but by following this structure you will gain the most benefit and greatly reduce the possibility of injuries.

The first stage is dynamic stretches. Slowly increase in movement and intensity for approximately ten minutes. This will stimulate your respiratory and circulatory systems, leading into aerobic-style exercise, which should be the start of your main program. Increase the range of movement with one exercise flowing into the next and rotating between arms, legs, and core exercise.

The second stage is more intense. The type of exercises you do may vary depending on any injury, an illness, or your fitness level. Do not let age be a barrier to giving most exercises a try. All fast-moving exercises are okay. These may include running on the spot. Or, remember the star jump from your youth? Sometimes these are called jumping jacks. You jump up in the air, extending your arms and legs when you are off the ground.

The third stage is "high-intensity, short-interval training," otherwise known as HISIT, plus aerobics sessions. Both are essential if you are looking to achieve weight loss. HISIT is designed to increase your heart rate for short intervals then to lower it for a short period and repeat this time and time again. This will get your metabolism working for you, burning fat. For example, this can be done on a stationary exercise bike. Pedal as hard as you can for eight seconds, then pedal lightly for twelve seconds (twenty seconds in all). Do this three times (which makes one minute). These time intervals are easy to track. Once you have been going for a few minutes, you will realize what a great routine it is. It is harder work than it sounds. If you do not have a bike, try running on the spot then walking for the same time periods. In fact, this method can be adapted to most free-flowing exercises. You can change the time periods depending on the degree of difficulty. The aerobic and HISIT sessions together should equal approximately thirty minutes.

The fourth state should be a slowing down in intensity, a ten-minute session of weight resistance plus exercises using less body movement. A great exercise to finish up on and lead into static stretching is the plank. Now it is time to relax and stretch for approximately ten minutes.

To review:

Warm-up = ten minutes
Aerobic = fifteen minutes (small hydration—two mouthfuls, approximately 100 millilitres or half a cup)
HISIT = fifteen minutes (small hydration)
Weights = ten minutes (small hydration)
Stretching = ten minutes (small hydration)
Total = one hour

Relax and have a good drink of water; you don't have to be sweating to require extra hydration.

This session was designed with weight loss in mind. If you are happy with your weight or you have reached your goal weight but you would like to increase your fitness level, this is a good program also. If your weight is not an issue and your fitness is not a problem because you are already walking, playing tennis, golf, or participating in other activities, or if you have an existing medical condition, you can modify the program. In this case the warm-up and static stretching stay the same. You can alter the main body of the program to include more weight resistance as well as balance and coordination exercises at a more leisurely pace.

Isometric Exercise (muscles don't move, but they work!)

Isometric exercise is a form of exercise in which muscles are engaged or tensed but have no movement or change in length. You hold your own body weight, an added weight, or you have resistance without movement. Good results can be achieved without equipment and in a short time frame. The plank is an example. Or try pushing against a wall.

Why not do isometric exercises and nothing else? The answer is that there is no movement in isometric exercise, and movement is good for coordination, balance, and speed. Our muscles would lose an amount of elasticity without movement. Isometric exercises are too beneficial not to include them, and should be done before, or incorporated into, static stretching. They can be worked into your main program. One way is to hold your pose or position for a few seconds when your muscles are under load.

Regular Exercise

Regular exercise increases the production of endorphins in your brain, giving you that "feel good feeling." Exercise also increases muscle strength and flexibility, lowers inflammation, and lubricates the joints, which can stimulate better joint function. This can help with chronic joint pain, and if continued, can promote temporary ongoing or even permanent relief.

Regular exercise as we grow older is incredibly important to maintain our quality of life. One of the major concerns as we age is having a fall and breaking our bones. Weight and resistance training will maintain and possibly improve bone density, which will increase your chances of not breaking bones if you are unfortunate enough to have a fall.

Aerobic-style training with plenty of movement will help you with your balance and coordination; it makes you more agile and flexible, conditions that could possibly prevent a fall.

Strong back muscles can help support your body. And remember, a strong core = a stable back.

With good posture and toned muscles, you are going to look and feel great.

Compare Exercise Machines

If you are thinking of buying an expensive exercise machine, here are a few things to think about. You could pay the same price for a long-term gym membership. If you join a gym for the same amount of money, you will have the choice of many exercise machines to use. There is a lot of competition between gyms, and your membership can be affordable with a no-contract, pay-as-you-go option. Additionally, the social aspect of a gym can by encouraging and fun!

If you do decide you would rather do a workout in the privacy of your own home, let us compare the most popular machines.

Treadmill

If you decide a treadmill is for you, then correct use is essential. They are great for burning calories. And they are great if the weather is inclement. But they can be boring; an outside walk to me is much better. Remember to always wear a safety stop device, as the machine will keep moving if you have a fall, and if this happens, you can sustain serious injuries.

Here are some tips for using a treadmill:

- Stay upright—no looking down.
- Do not over stride.
- Do not hunch your shoulders.
- Walk heel to toe.
- Bend your arms at 90 degrees.
- Relax your shoulders.
- Keep most arm motion in back of your body.
- Keep your arm motion opposite your leg motion, and at the same speed.

Cross-Trainer, or Elliptical Machine

With this sort of machine, you work both your arms and legs at the same time. The action is very gentle on your joints. This, again, is a good way to burn calories. Always keep good upright posture.

Stationary Bike

Bike workouts are great for burning calories. It is easy to vary speed and load, easy on your joints, great for your legs, but your arms still need a workout.

Most important, whether you use an upright or a recumbent bike, is correct use. Keep good seating posture, your back straight, and your shoulders back. Adjust the seat distance from pedals so your knees remain "soft" (with a slight bend) when the pedals have reached the bottom of the stroke.

Rowing Machine

This has to be my favourite. Rowing works most, if not all, of your major muscle groups. Rowing machines have a great action that is easy on your joints.

If you are thinking about buying only one exercise machine, the rowing machine is a "no brainer."

Tips on using a rowing machine:

- Keep your back straight.
- Do not hunch your shoulders.
- Keep good heel contact, and drive back through your legs.
- Keep your knees and elbows soft (with a slight bend); never lock them up.
- Use a fluid movement; avoid a jerking action.

Note: I have not reviewed the cable weight–type apparatus, as they can be quite bulky, and not everyone has the space, but if you have room in your garage, they are great for maintaining bone density.

Free Weights versus Machines

Simple free weights can give you more freedom of movement in your exercises than machines can give. Combine them together for a great work out.

Thinking of Joining a Gym?

Here is some advice and tips on gyms and gym etiquette.

- If you feel you are overweight, don't worry about your body shape. Don't compare yourself to others. You won't be the only overweight person there, of course. People will admire you for deciding to do something about it. Keep thinking of how you are going to look in the future when you have achieved weight loss.

- It is a good idea, if possible, to join with a friend or maybe a family member. This may make you feel more at ease. Also, you can encourage and help each other!

- Always take two small towels with you. One is for your personal use and the other is for the equipment. Wipe down the equipment after use whether you are perspiring or not. Some gyms supply disinfectant wipes or spray cleaner and paper towels to be used for this purpose.

- Keep hydrated. Take at least one litre of water with you. Hydration helps with fatigue and flushes toxins from your body.

- Do not eat a big meal before a gym session, as digestion will make you lethargic. Having a light snack or a protein shake is ideal.

- Turn your mobile phone off and relax.

- Wear appropriate clothing—not too light or too loose.

- Do not do all cardio. Use the treadmill or bike to warm up and burn calories. Do not be afraid to use the other equipment. Instructions are usually printed on the side or front of each machine. Gym staff members are there to help. Most people in a gym are more than willing to help; they love it. I never offer advice outside my own gym, but I love it if I am asked for it. I take it as a compliment.

- It is a good idea to have a few sessions with a personal trainer, just to start you off on the right track. A trainer can help you make sure your posture and technique are correct, and can give you tips that will help prevent any injuries from occurring.

- Every muscle is important and has a purpose, so build and tone as many as you can at each session.

- Balance your session as you move from one apparatus to another. Work your legs, arms, and core for a short period then come back and repeat. This way, while you are working one part of your body, the other parts can rest.

- Gradually increase size of weights, intensity, reps, and sets.

- Replace all the equipment you have used.
- Do not hog a certain piece of equipment, especially if it is the only one in the gym.
- If you do have a training buddy, be competitive and keep a chart on how you are doing. You can feed off your training buddy's energy if you hit a wall.
- Most important of all is to be patient and increase your time, intensity, and workload gradually.

Things Not to Do when You Start an Exercise Program of Any Kind

- Don't stop your non-exercise physical activity. Add your exercise program to your normal daily routine. You will lose most of the benefit of the workout if you then spend the rest of the day resting on the lounge.
- Your workout should be intense and challenging, but don't make it so difficult that you are completely overwhelmed, muscle sore, and exhausted. Remember that you will need to feel refreshed and ready for another session twenty-four to forty-eight hours later.
- Don't go straight into a hard program without a good warm up even if you are short on time. Doing so could cause an injury that could set you back for months.
- Don't try to make up for lost time. If you miss a session, don't try to double up on your next session. Remember that a slow, consistent, gradual approach will prevent overload.
- Don't do the same exercise program at each session. Avoid getting into a rut. Keep yourself fresh so you can look forward to every session.
- Don't skip a session because of lack of time. A full twenty-minute session is better than nothing. Increase the intensity, but do not miss your warm up even if it does use up half of your time. A warm up is movement, and all movement is beneficial.
- Don't expect too much too quickly. Stick with a gradual and consistent approach. If you push yourself too hard, you risk losing correct posture, which can lead to a painful injury.

- Don't push yourself so hard that you lose interest and end up putting physical exercise in the too-hard basket.
- Don't expect miracles if you are trying to lose weight. Safe and sustainable weight loss is a half a kilogram (about one pound) per week, and you may experience a weight-loss plateau.
- Don't exercise close to bedtime. Activity will put your mind in a highly active state, making it less likely that you will be able to fall asleep quickly.
- Don't look for big, sweeping changes. Consistency is more important than short-term unsustainable gains. Don't let your age limit your expectations, but do set realistic goals for your ability.

Things You Should Do in Any Exercise Program

- Be conscious of your posture 24/7.
- If you spend most of your working hours behind a desk, go for a short walk around the office (or outdoors!) whenever you can. This should be at least every two hours, and more often if possible. Try standing at your desk even if only for short periods, or do some chair squats (stand up sit down repeatedly). Go for a walk during lunchtime; not only is it good exercise, it may clear your mind. Make your weekends active ones.
- Remember to squat when picking objects off the floor; this is great for your legs and easy on your back.
- Think of ways to work exercise moves into your everyday routine. Squats, lunges, and short walks can be done while you are talking on the phone. Do some squats while you hang out the washing. Use the kitchen bench to do some incline push-ups while you wait for the microwave. Think of all that wasted time during commercial breaks on television!
- Challenge yourself, set yourself targets, and make a list of what you want to achieve. The list will keep your mind in the right place and give you purpose. Believe in yourself, think positively, and keep mentally strong. Challenging yourself will help prevent a plateau. A plateau occurs when you level off and cease making gains.

- Use the mirror to motivate yourself. If you do not like what you see, keep working at it. The best motivator I know is seeing muscles you did not know you had! You'll like what you see!
- Training with a friend can make you both more accountable. You don't want to let the other person down, so you turn up for a session you might have otherwise skipped. The other person probably felt the same way! Turning up can sometimes be challenging, but just turning up makes you a winner! The feeling of well-being you will achieve from working towards your goals makes the effort well worth it.
- Increase your water intake. Keeping your body well hydrated will help with muscle growth and recovery.
- Start using the stairs instead of the lift during non-exercise parts of your day.
- Get off the lounge and out of your comfort zone. The rewards are great. Live life to the fullest.
- To prevent boredom in your exercise program, add variety by trying new exercises and varying the intensity and duration of the ones that are most familiar to you.
- Sometimes you may need a break to recuperate, especially if you work out most days at an intense level.
- No matter how, when, or where you train, try to close the door on the rest of the world and make every training session your space.

Smile – it reduces stress!

Think positively!

Celebrate small successes!

Don't put off starting. You may never start if you procrastinate. Whenever possible, try to exercise in the morning. You are more likely to stick at a routine. Getting motivated for an afternoon session after a hard and possibly stressful morning may be difficult.

LET'S LOOK AT SOME COMMON PROBLEM AREAS

The exercises in this book are meant to complement sensible, commonsense, healthy eating habits. Consult your health care provider for more information on good nutrition.

If you have excess fat anywhere in your body, you need to do some cardio/aerobic work as part of your session. This will start the fat-burning process, and the non-aerobic exercises will tone and firm your muscles.

Ladies

Excess fat at the back of your upper arms (tricep area) is commonly called "bingo wings" or "tuckshop arms." You need to target these muscles at each session, as they are not used often in your normal daily activity. The best exercises are tricep dips and tricep extension.

Fat on your back is made to look worse by bra straps. You cannot see it without looking in a mirror, so you tend to forget it is there. It can be seen by others. If you wish to look good in that summer dress, you need to start in the winter. If you go to a gym, look for the lat pull-down apparatus. Exercises you can do at home for your back are standing (or on-your-knees) push ups, opposite arm, opposite leg, or superman pose. These are all great.

'Does my "bum" look big in these jeans?' This is an easy one. Squats and lunges are perfect; doing both will work all your glutes top and bottom.

Fat around your waist? Burn, burn, burn! Plenty of cardio/aerobic work, then core exercises, sit-ups, and the plank will work well.

Extra weight on your thighs! More burn, then squats and lunges are standard. Add side lunges, which are the same as normal lunges, but off to the side. Also stand holding the back of a chair or similar furniture for balance, then come up onto the ball of your left foot, engage your abs.

Keeping your hips facing forward, simply swing your right leg across your left and back. Do ten reps then alternate legs.

Men

There is one huge problem that hangs over your belt buckle, commonly known as a "beer belly." It is a combination of too much food, the wrong food, and inactivity. Beer to excess only adds to the problem. Throw in a set of man boobs, and there we have it. I know plenty of fit, active men in a healthy weight range who enjoy a few beers in moderation, including myself.

The answer is to move as much as you can. Start walking wherever possible. For short trips, leave the car at home or in the car park.

It takes a long time to acquire the extra weight, and it also takes time to get you back to a healthy weight, but the results can be life changing.

The quickest way to burn fat with exercise is to eat less sugar. Your body will normally burn sugar as one of its first energy sources, so it stands to reason if you have less sugar in your diet, your exercise program will start burning fat faster. You cannot target a specific part of your body for fat reduction. Your body burns fat indiscriminately. Unfortunately, belly fat will probably be the last reserve to begin to move. But no one is going to do it for you. Also remember that muscle weighs more than fat, so you could be turning fat into muscle even though the scales are telling you that you're gaining weight.

When you are ready to start exercising burn, burn, burn with aerobic-style exercise to stimulate your circulatory and respiratory systems. Slowly advance to harder and more intense workouts. All movement is good.

BENEFITS OF LOOKING GOOD AND FEELING FIT

Try to think of your new lifestyle changes as a consistent improvement as you go forward towards a new life that you can sustain and enjoy. If you work hard on your fitness and health, there must be rewards. Your age should not be a barrier to doing whatever it is you want to. There is nothing wrong with feeling good about yourself, walking into a room with confidence, knowing that you look good without taking yourself to seriously.

Here are a few words of encouragement to help you get through the hard work:

- You will experience the joy of pain-free movement and the freedom that it can provide.
- You will perform everyday chores with ease, and do them better than most people your age.
- You will be among the most active people in your age group— only those in the top 10 percent are active!
- You will be able to continue longer in the work force if you wish to.
- You will perform better at your chosen sport.
- You will be envied and admired by your friends.
- You will play harder and sleep better.
- You will look fabulous in your favourite clothing styles and size.
- You will live longer.
- Because you will have strong muscles and bones, you will limit your chances of having a fall, and limit the chance of injury if you do have a fall or an accident.
- You will enjoy an overall better quality of life.
- Exercise will improve your moods and help reduce stress, anxiety, and depression.

- Exercise will reduce the risk of many diseases.
- You will be better able to cope with life's challenges.

If you wish to be truly happy and you hope to have a long and fruitful life with fulfilment through your own effort you have to give your life meaning and purpose, a purpose outside of your own self interest.

Find your purpose and get more out of life!

EXPLANATION

Active Rest	*Low energy movement*
Aerobic	*Moderate to hard activity at a fast pace*
Bone Density	*The amount of bone mineral in bone tissue*
Compound	*Two or more actions involved making the exercise more difficult*
Diabetes	*Your body's ability to use sugar is impaired* • *Type One: Rare and requires Insulin injection* • *Type Two: More common and can be managed with regular activity and health eating habits.*
Dynamic	*Energy force in action. Plenty of movement*
Hyrdration	*Keeping plenty of water in your body*
Isometric	*No movement involved*
1 Kilo	*= 2.2 pound*
Posture	*The position of your body and limbs*
Repetition	*The number an exercise is repeated*
Static	*Stationary*
Structuring	*Planning and arranging*
Technique	*The method or procedure used to perform an exercise*

Now you have read my book….

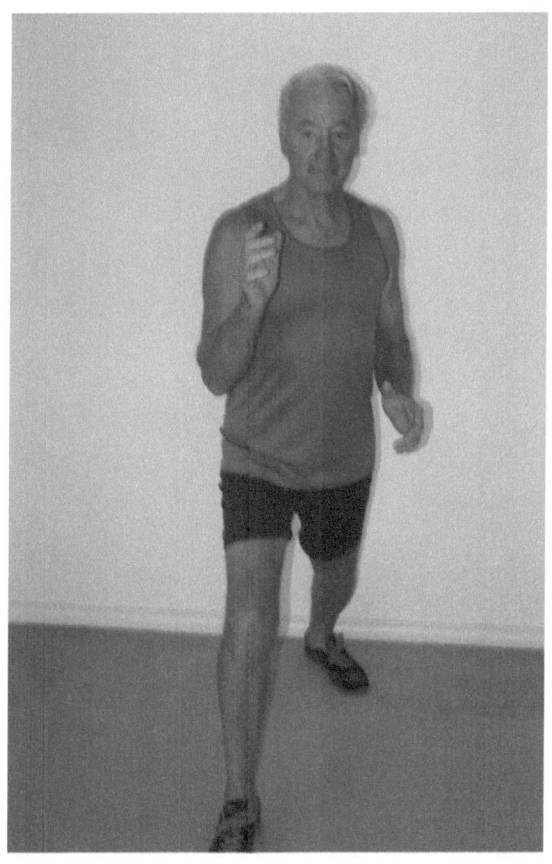

Now its up to you to turn the page and start your new lifestyle.